APPLYING ALCOHOLICS ANONYMOUS PRINCIPLES TO THE DISEASE OF RACISM

APPLYING ALCOHOLICS ANONYMOUS PRINCIPLES TO THE DISEASE OF RACISM

Kenneth L. Radcliffe

To order additional copies of this book, contact:
Kenneth L. Radcliffe Services
www.theisaiahproject.name
or
Xlibris Corporation
1-888-795-4274
www.Xlibris.com
Orders@Xlibris.com
89698

Contents

Applying Alcoholics Anonymous Principles
To The Disease Of Racism

This book is based on a paper, Applying AA (Alcoholics Anonymous)
Principles to the Disease of Racism, that was originally written and
submitted in partial completion of the requirements for the
Training Program on Alcoholism and Chemical Dependency
Counseling, Rockland Council on
Alcoholism and Other Drug Dependence Inc. in June 1994 by the author
Kenneth L. Radcliffe

Revised November 2, 2011

*To my wife Shirley, daughters, Kendahl, Lisa, grandsons Elijah, Justin,
and family, thank you.*

*To the Church and a special group of Men and Women of Faith who have
helped me on this path. Thank You.*

*To Sandy Bernabei of the AntiRacist Alliance, Ron Chisom,
David Billings and Margery Freeman of the People's Institute;
Robert "Bob" Gangi, Dr. Barbara Wallace, Black Men, Men of Color
(MOC), Black Women, Women Of Color (WOC), Jackie Rowe-Adams,
Gabriel Sayegh, Goodie and Jeanette Goudeau, Fr. Ben Taylor,
The Correctional Association of New York, Thank You.*

This Book is dedicated to the Memory of Kathleen Moran

Introduction

*"Racial tensions and conflicts between groups are due
primarily to issues of power, privilege and control . . ."*[1]

*Segregation, discrimination, bias, prejudice, bigotry, separation, apartheid,
racism, double standard, partiality,* and *equality* are terms used in the course
of daily living. In a word, the sun never seems to set without a person or
persons experiencing through sight, sound, thought, feeling, or opinion
some one or a multiple of these words. They are expressed, experienced,
or encountered in most aspects of the American society, whether in
our interpersonal relationships at home, on the job, in academia, the
marketplace, or experienced and interpreted for us through media, print
and electronic.

Racism, it can be said, is one of the major issues of the day—past
New York City mayoral elections, the elections in South Africa, the racial
strife in Rwanda, the "ethnic cleansing" in Sarajevo, the strife in Israel,
and we should not exclude the continued prosecution of the Nazis as a
result of their earlier attempts to annihilate the Jews. Another example
is the charges of anti-Semitism directed at Minister Louis Farrakhan
and the Nation of Islam several years ago. Charges and countercharges
of racism continue being hurled between groups: White People, Black
People, Jews, Muslims, etc.

---

[1]   Corsini, Raymond J., Ed., *International Encyclopedia of Psychiatry, Psychology,
Psychoanalysis and Neurology,* Wiley Inter Science Publications, p.39.

Rationale

The purpose of this book will be threefold. First, it will seek to demonstrate that racism is a disease, a mental illness. Its symptoms are similar to those of the disease of alcoholism. Second, that racism like alcoholism has not been proven curable at this point in time. However, like alcoholism, it is treatable. The symptoms can be arrested! A treatment plan for the victims of racism, primarily African Americans and other peoples of color living on the North American continent will be suggested and why. Because the lives of these victims of racism, like the lives of those affected by the behavior of the alcoholic in most instances, are dysfunctional. Finally the origin and role of the Black Church's resistance to racism in America will be described briefly.

In order to accomplish this task, the structure of this paper will be as follows:

I.   A Brief History: The Evolution of Racism
    A. Definition of terms
       1. What is racism?
       2. Who is a racist?
II. Racism is a Disease
III. Applying Alcoholics Anonymous Principles to the Disease of Racism
    Comparisons/Similarities to Alcoholism
IV. Why Racism Should Be of Concern to Clinicians and Individuals Who
    Aspire to Counsel Others in the Areas of Alcohol, Drug, and Other
    Substance Abuse/Addictions
V. The Black Church; Source of the Africans' Strength Then and Now

I

A Brief History

We begin the brief history with a few references from the following historical sources. Dr. Brewton Berry, in his book, *Race Relations,"—Interaction of Ethnic and Racial Groups,* states that the system of racism as we know and experience it today evolved slowly out of the institution of slavery, introduced first by the Portuguese in their own country and later on the continent of America as a source of labor.[2] The Spanish were not long in following in order to meet the growing European demand for sugar and rum, which was being harvested abundantly in the virgin Americas and the Caribbean.

Lerone Bennett, Jr. in his book, *Before the Mayflower,* writes, "Spaniards who took the lead in the exploration attempted at first to enslave Indians. But they died so fast that Bishop Bartolome de Las Casas, a famous missionary, recommended in 1517 the importation of Africans, a recommendation he lived to regret. The development of large-scale plantations created a demand for men that casual kidnapping could not supply. In the wake of that development, the vision of European monarchs shifted and the African-European dialogue became a monologue focused almost exclusively on a trade in men. Within a few years, hundreds of thousands of blacks were crossing the Atlantic each year, and the soil of Africa and America was drenched with their blood. 'Strange,' said Eric Williams, 'that an article like sugar, so sweet and necessary to human existence, should have occasioned such crimes and bloodshed.'[3]

---

[2]   Berry, Brewton, PhD. *"Race Relations -Interaction of Ethnic and Racial Groups,* Houghton Mifflin Co. Boston, Ma., 1951. p. 45.

[3]   Bennett, Lerone Jr., *Before the Mayflower,* Johnson publishing Co. Inc. Chicago, Ill, p. 34.

The Dutch, England, and France were soon in hot pursuit, exploring the New World and exploiting Africa, urged on by the vast fortunes being made by Portugal and Spain from their sugar, tobacco, and coffee plantations in Central and South America. Basil Davidson in his book, *The African Slave Trade,* explains, "The explanations were twofold: Sugar and tobacco planting. Sugar had been rare in Europe. Now it was big business. For many European merchants the rest of the seventeenth century was literally the century of sugar. Tobacco became important, and so did rum and West Indian coffee and cotton. But the grand consumer of slaves in the new lands across the Atlantic, and the great maker of profits for Europe was King Sugar. Neither sugar nor tobacco could be grown without abundant field labour."[4]

The Feudal System of Europe Is Transported to Early North America

Unlike Portugal and Spain, England had its own internal system of labor: the indentured servant. Thomas F. Gossett writes in *Race: The History of an Idea in America,* "The fact that the legal condition of the first Negroes who arrived in America was no different from that of white bond servants . . ."[5] Bennett agrees. "But the first black immigrants (Antoney and Isabella and the Jamestown group) were not slaves. This is a fact of critical importance in the history of Black America. They came, these first Blacks, in the same way that most of the first white immigrants came—under duress and pressure. They found a system (indentured servitude) which enabled poor whites to come to America and sell their services for a stipulated number of years, to planters. Under this system thousands of whites—paupers, ne'er-do-wells, religious dissenters, waifs, prisoners and prostitutes—were shipped to the colonies and sold to the highest bidder. Many were sold as the first Blacks were sold, by the captains of the ships. Some were kidnapped on the streets of London and Bristol, as the first Blacks were kidnapped in the villages of Africa."[6]

---

[4] Davidson, Basil, *The African Slave Trade,* Back Bay Books, Boston, Ma., p.75.

[5] Gossett, Thomas F., *Race: The History of an Idea in America*, Southern Methodist University Press, Dallas, Tx., 1963, p. 30.

[6] Bennett, Lerone Jr., *Before the Mayflower,* Johnson publishing Co. Inc. Chicago, Ill, p. 35.

Race and Color Not an Issue Yet

Gossett, "The Negroes were pushed into a society where most of the people were bond servants and therefore to some degree unfree. Since the word slave had no meaning in English law, the Negro was thought of as a servant and not as a slave. *The fact that no time for the ending of the Negroe's servitude was set is no proof that Negroes really were considered as slaves,'* argues Handlin. The reason was that, in England, there was a plentiful labor supply, *the employer was accustomed to a system in which the expiration of a term of service had little meaning because the servant was nearly always obliged by his circumstances simply to sign up for another term of service."*[7]

Color and race were not an issue yet in the development of early America. Gossett, "There is evidence however that there was a caste barrier between whites and Negroes before the institution of slavery legally came into being. Guy B. Johnson observes that it is extremely doubtful whether white people of the colonies felt the same toward Negroes as they did toward their white bond servants."[8] Bennett agrees, "In Virginia then, as in other colonies, the first Black settlers fell into a well established socio-economic groove which carried with it *no implications of racial inferiority.* That came later."[9]

Bennett continues, "Working in the same fields, sharing the same huts, the same situation, and the same grievances, the first black and white Americans, aristocrats excepted, developed strong bonds of sympathy and mutuality. They ran away together, played together, and revolted together. They mated and married, siring a sizable mixed population.

In the process, the black and white servants—the majority of the colonial population—created a racial wonderland that seems somehow un-American in its lack of obsession with race and color. There was, to be sure, prejudice then, but it was largely English class prejudice, which was distributed without regard to race, creed, or color. There was also, needless to say, prejudiced individuals in the colony, but—and *this is the fundamental difference between prejudice and racism*—their personal quirks and obsessions were not focused and directed by the organized

---

[7.] Gossett, Thomas F., *Race: The History of an Idea in America*, Southern Methodist University Press, Dallas, Tx., 1963, p. 29.

[8.] Ibid, p. 30.

[9.] Bennett, Lerone Jr., *Before the Mayflower*, Johnson publishing Co. Inc. Chicago, Ill, p. 35.

will of a community. The basic division at that juncture was between servants and free people, and there were whites and blacks on both sides of the line.

Of all the improbable aspects of this situation, the oddest—to modern blacks and whites—is that white people did not seem to know that they were white. It appears from surviving evidence that the first white colonists had no concept of themselves as white people. The legal documents identified whites as Englishmen and/or Christians. The word *white*, with its burden of arrogance and biological pride, developed late in the century, as a direct result of slavery and the organized debasement of blacks.

The same point can be made from the other side of the line. For a long time in America, there was no legal name to focus white anxiety. The first blacks were called blackamoors, moors, negers and negars. The word *Negro*, a Spanish and Portuguese term for black, did not come into general use in Virginia until the latter part of the century."[10]

Gradually, the status of the African began to change. Note the following comments. Gossett, "The labor system in the colonies tended to work to the advantage of the white bond-servant. In order to combat the publicity given to harsh treatment of servants in the colonies, *the term of indentured service was shortened, first for Englishmen and later on for Irishmen and other aliens. The Negro on the other hand did not have to be placated in this way because there was no need to encourage more Negroes to come to the colonies or to combat adverse opinion in Africa.* As the term of service for white bond-servants was decreasing, the demand for labor was increasing. In these circumstances, the number of Negroes imported greatly increased."[11]

The Early American Dream Becomes a Nightmare for Others

For a while, it would seem that America was truly the land of opportunity for all those who arrived. Bennett, "In the interim, a period of forty years or more the first Black settlers accumulated land, voted, testified in court, mingled with the whites on the basis of equality. They owned other Black

---

[10] *Ibid.* p.40.

[11] Gossett, Thomas F., *Race: The History of an Idea in America,* Southern Methodist University Press, Dallas, Tx., 1963, pp. 29, 30.

servants, and certain Blacks imported and paid for white servants whom they apparently held in servitude."[12]

However, the position of the Africans in America would change radically, a change that would, two hundred years later, rend this country asunder. Gossett, "In the 1660's the status of Negroes was finally recognized as different from other servants. The Maryland House enacted a bill which stated, 'All Negroes and other slaves shall serve Durante Vita.' Virginia law was at first more indirect. In an act of 1661 imposing penalties on runaways, it recognized that some Negroes were to be slaves for life. It was not until 1670 that Virginia laws specified that 'all servants not Christians' who were brought into the colony by sea were to be slaves for life."[13]

Over one hundred years later, these two regional laws were ratified and incorporated into the bylaws of the new Republic of America. Thus, racism made its way into the constitutional convention in Philadelphia in 1787. Inserted were three clauses that would turn this great document from a great blessing to a curse. The conveners agreed in writing to count three-fifths of a state's slave population in apportioning representation, to forbid Congress from ending the slave trade until 1808, and to require that fugitive slaves who cross state lines be surrendered to their owners. This legal ratification, reducing Africans to property, a thing, engineered so skillfully by a few white Anglo-Saxon Protestant (WASP) men and two Roman Catholics (gentlemen farmers and plantation owners), became the law of the land.

Their political maneuvering and conviction carried the day in that it was not only their legal right but now their God-given moral right to dominate, subdue, dehumanize, and conquer other human beings, especially since those people did not look, think, act, or choose like them. The system of racism as we know and experience to this very day in America, evolved out of man's greed for money, power, privilege and prestige. It was a man-made organized legal system enslaving other men, women, and children, robbing them of their humanity, mutual heritage, and labor in order to satisfy his own addictions in his quest for riches by supplying old-world (Western Europe) markets' newfound addictions: sugar made into rum (alcohol), West Indian coffee and tea (caffeine), and tobacco (nicotine).

---

12. Bennett, Lerone Jr., *Before the Mayflower,* Johnson Publishing Co. Inc. Chicago, Ill, p. 35

13. Gossett, Thomas F., Race: *The History of an Idea in America,* Southern Methodist University Press, p. 30

Author's Note; It is alleged that Bishop de Las Casas before he died, regretted* recommending to King Charles of Spain in 1517 that African slaves replace the Amerindians as a labor source. His reason for the recommendation was to stop the mass annihilation of the native Indians who he cared and advocated for. Their population was rapidly diminishing due to many factors, bodies weaken by forced labor and diseases brought by the Europeans. An estimated 2 million had died from a small pox epidemic that began in 1516.* There was mass suicide and mass infanticide. The Africans he suggested were stronger and better able to function in the agricultural conditions of the Americas. The King acting on his suggestion gave impetus to what was to become man's greatest act of horror and inhumanity to his fellow human beings, the lucrative African slave trade.**

Sources: *Thomas Clarkson and the Abolition of Slavery, Background Information, Section 1 from the Teachers Resource Pack for KS1-4 written by Maureen James, B.Ed.(Hons), M.A. for the Wisebech & Fenland Museum, UK, 2007, p.3.
     **Berry, Brewton, PhD., Race Relations—Interaction of Ethnic and Racial Groups, Houghton Mifflin Co. Boston, Ma., 1951. p. 45
     Author's Note; (Some Scholars estimate that of the 40 - 55 million African slaves transported by the Europeans to the Americas, only 10-15 million of them survived the journey. Africans sent to Brazil, were about 4 million alone. The Arabs transported about 17 million Africans to the Middle East. Sources: "The Slave Trade", Hugh Thomas, 1997; "The Origins of the African Slave Trade, Back to History," Piero Scaruffi).

Slavery in America Was Made Unique

One could say "Slavery, so what?" Slavery has existed since man has been on this planet, and historians will agree. However, slavery, once introduced to the virgin Americas was unique. The following comments will help to demonstrate what made American slavery especially unique and drastically different from that form of slavery that already existed.

Bennett, "There was a crucial difference, however, between ancient slavery and modern slavery. Ancient slavery, which had little or nothing to do with race, was justified primarily by the rules of war. Christians and Moslems added new dimensions to this ancient institution, capturing and enslaving one another for religious reasons. The same rationale served both groups when economic interests and improved technology focused attention on Africa."[14]

Slavery, it has sometimes been argued, was first considered as an interim institution designed to convert both Negroes and Indians to Christianity. Gossett, "It is interesting, however, that among the colonists of the seventeenth and eighteenth centuries, it is the heathenism of the Negroes and Indians rather than their race that is emphasized as a basis for their enslavement. In 1710, Cotton Mather founded a school for slaves. While admitting that the slave trade is "a spectacle that shocks humanity," he wondered whether the Negroes coming to this country might not represent the obscure workings of Providence. *'God, whom you must remember to be "your Master in heaven," has brought them, and put them into your hands. Who can tell what good he has brought them for? How if they could be the elect of God, fetched from Africa, or the Indies, and brought into your families, on purposes, that by the means of their being there, they may be brought home unto the Shepherd of souls!'*

In the South, when the institution of slavery came under heavy attack during the nineteenth century, a principle justification offered for it was a means of converting the heathen. In the eighteenth century however, when slavery was virtually unchallenged in the South, we find very little reliance upon this particular argument. At least Bishop Berley testified in 1731 that American slaveholders had "an *irrational contempt'* of the blacks as creatures of another species, who had no right to be instructed or admitted to the sacraments."[15]

A Prototype of the Racist System Emerges

The following describes the early developmental stages of a distorted thought process that was to be brutally enforced for the next two hundred years. Joel Kovel in his book, *White Racism: A Psychohistory*, takes us into what could have been the mindset of a slaver of the period. He writes. "A particular relationship developed under specific circumstances of American history. Although there were points of similarity with other slave systems, much of which remain the subject of active investigation, a basic and characteristically American style emerged as Black slavery hardened into

---

14.   Bennett, Lerone Jr., *Before the Mayflower,* Johnson publishing Co. Inc. Chicago, Ill.

15.   Gossett, Thomas F., *Race: The History Of an Idea in America,* Southern Methodist University Press, Dallas, Tx., 1963, p. 31

an *institution*. The slaver in effect said to his slave, *'while I own much, much more than my body, you own not even your body: your body shall be detached from yourself and yourself shall thereby be reduced to subhuman status. And being detached and kept alive, your body shall serve me in many ways: by work on my capitalist plantations to extract the most that can be taken from the land in the cheapest and therefore most rational manner; as a means to my bodily pleasure—both as a nurse to my children and as a female body for sexual use (for my own women are somehow deficient in this regard); and as a medium of exchange, salable like any other commodity of exchange along with or separate from the bodies of your family. For in fact you have no family, since a family is a system that pertains to human beings and you are not human. And since I, being a man of the West, value things which are owned above all else, I hold you—or, rather, the owned part of you, your body—in very high regard and wish to retain you as my property forever. On the other hand, since I have a certain horror of what I am doing and since you are the living reminder of this horror and are subhuman to boot, I am horrified by you, disgusted by you, and wish to have nothing to do with you, wish, in fact to be rid of you. And since this set of ideas is inconsistent and will stand neither the test of reason nor of my better values, going to distort it, spit it up. and otherwise defend myself against the realization.'*

In practice this schema underwent endless variations. The distillation of this notion was the essence of the American slave system however, and had a reality of its own: it became the basis in [our] *culture* of the *idea* of the black man, and it has consequently become the historical nucleus of our present-day racism."[16] As H. Rap Brown, a black revolutionary of the early 1970s, said, "*Racism is as American as Mom and apple pie*" (see exhibit 1).

The African Is Reduced to a Thing—Property

While the WASP included his own kind initially, to the exclusion of Catholics; the Irish; and later the Italians, the Jews, the Middle Eastern Europeans, and the Asians, only the African was legally dehumanized in the pursuit of the American dream—his manifest destiny. The African became property, a thing. A man being made property was made to appear rational. Kovel describes this development. "Property is some portion of the external

---

16. Kovel, Joel *White Racism: A Psychohistory* Pantheon Books, New York, A division of Random House, 1970, pp. 18, 19.

world that a man's self may call its own. Property means therefore that a man's self—the inner idea of his personage—is united and enlarged by part of the "thing"—world. One part of the world ordinarily owned by every man's self is his own body. Indeed, the body is really all of the world that the self can own—ordinarily. But the West is extraordinary in that it has held for centuries that the summum bonum of life on earth is the expansion of the self through its acquisition of property.

On the other hand, the West, which was to convulse the globe in its search for material acquisitions, has never really been happy with its desire for property. Nowadays the whole process—desire for and horror of acquisition—has, without losing its basic force *been rationalized* and *made abstract*: this has been the consistent direction of our history."[17]

Kovel continues. "We noted earlier that property rationally begins and ends with the possession of one's own body. It was precisely this limit that the West *breached with its slavery*. For the American slaver did not simply own the *body* of his black slave—although even that may have been more extreme than some earlier variants of slavery, where the slave's freedom was but limited and only his work owned. The American slaver went one step further in cultural development: he first reduced the human self of his black slave to a body and then reduced the body to *a thing; he dehumanized his slave, and made him quantifiable*; and thereby absorbed him into a rising *world market of productive exchange*. In the creation of this world market, the Westerner was changing his entire view of reality—and changing reality in accordance with his new conception of it. Thus in the new culture of the West, the black human was reduced to a *black thing*, virtually the same in certain key aspects as the rest of non-human nature—all of which could become property"[18] (see exhibits 1 & 4).

C. Eric Lincoln in his book, *Race, Religion and the Continuing American Dilemma*, writes. "In those colonies where slaves were considered indispensable to the plantation economy, the economic investment in human bodies was enormous, and the planters were suspicious of any tampering with their property rights. Talk to a planter about the soul of a Negro, commented a writer in a popular colonial journal, "and he'll apt to tell you that the body of one Negro may be worth 20 pounds, but the souls of a hundred of them would not yield him one farthing."[19] Kovel states

---

17. Ibid pp 16, 17.

18. Ibid p.18.

19. Lincoln, C. Eric, *Race, Religion and the Continuing American Dilemma*, Hill and Wang, New York, 1984, p.42.

further, "Of all America's exclusions, none approaches in strength that of the black people by white people, the distinction of a self and an other according to the mysterious quality of race, especially as revealed in the mark of skin color. Nothing looms quite so large, both as an endless crisis and as a sign of a deep cultural malaise, as does racism."[20]

Unlike the Spanish and the French, who were Catholic, the white Anglo-Saxon Protestants (WASP) viewed the black peon in a different light. Lincoln writes. "From the beginning the Anglo Americans considered the Blacks among them as beings of a lower order who, if they were human at all, were not human in the same sense that white men were human. Hence neither the blessings of liberty nor the comforts of heaven were considered to have any reference to Blacks. It was simply understood that 'men' meant *white* men, whether the context was social political, religious or general. In short, the American mindset was such as to effectively exclude Blacks from any frame of reference dealing with—what could be considered normative human interests or relations."[21]

There was also an economic theory. So decisive are the economic factors in the life of man that some scholars have looked to intergroup competition and exploitation for an understanding of race prejudice. O. C. Cox, one of the proponents of this idea, states, "Race prejudice is a social attitude propagated among the public by an exploiting class for the purpose of stigmatizing some groups as inferior so that the exploitation of either group itself or its resources may be justified."[22]

---

[20]. Kovel, Joel, *White Racism: A Psychohistory,* Pantheon Books, New York, A division of Random House, 1970, p.14.

[21]. Lincoln, C. Eric, *Race, Religion and the Continuing American Dilemma,* Hill and Wang, New York, 1984, p. 42.

[22]. Berry, Brewton, PhD., *Race Relations—Interaction of Ethnic and Racial Groups,* Houghton Mifflin Co. Boston Ma., 1951.

Racism Defined

Racism is not the following:

"Discrimination—(1) the act of discriminating or distinguishing differences; (2) the ability to make or perceive distinctions, perception, or discernment; (3) a showing of partiality or prejudice in treatment, action, or policies directed against minority groups.

Segregation—(1) a segregating or being segregated, specifically the policy or practice compelling racial groups to live apart from each other, go to separate schools, use separate social facilities, etc.; (2) genetics, the separation of allelic genes into different gametes during neurosis so that a particular gamete receives only one member of a pair of characters: See Mendel's Law.

Prejudice—a judgment of opinion made before the facts are known, preconceived idea, favorable or, more usually, unfavorable. (2a) A judgment of opinion held in disregard of facts that contradict it and unreasonable bias (a prejudice against modern art); (b) the holding of such judgments or opinions. (3) Suspicion, intolerance, or irrational hatred of other races, creeds, religions, occupations, etc. (4) Injury or harm resulting from some judgment or action of another or others—vt. diced-dicing: (1) to injure or harm as by some judgment or action and (2) to cause or show prejudice; bias—without prejudice: (1) without detriment or injury and (2) law without dismissal of or detriment to (a legal right, claim etc., often with to.

Bias (syn.—prejudice)—implies a preconceived and unreasonable judgment of opinion, usually an unfavorable one marked by suspicion, fear, or hatred (a murder motivated by race prejudice); bias implies a mental leaning in favor of or against someone or something [few of us are without bias of any kind]; partiality implies an inclination to favor a person or thing because of strong fondness or attachment [the conductor's partiality for the works of Brahms]; predilection implies a preconceived liking, formed as a result of one's background, temperament, etc., that inclines one to a particular preference [he has a predilection for murder mysteries].

Bigotry—the behavior, attitude or beliefs of a bigot; intolerance, prejudice.

Bigot—(1) a person who holds blindly and intolerantly to a particular creed, opinion, etc.; (2) a narrow-minded person."

Webster's New World Dictionary, Updated 1994 Edition, is the reference source that is used to define the above.

Racism as defined by the following sources:

"*Racism*—(1) is a belief or doctrine that inherent differences among various human races determine cultural or individual achievement, usually involving the idea that one's own race is superior and has a right to rule others. (2) A policy system of government, etc., based upon or fostering such a doctrine; discrimination. (3) Hatred or tolerance of another race or races."[23]

OR

"*Racism*—is the assumption that psychocultural traits and capacities are determined by biological race and that races differ decisively from one another, which is usually coupled with the belief in the inherent superiority of a particular race and its right to domination over others. (2a) A doctrine or political program based on the assumption of racism and designed to execute its principles. (2b) a political or social system founded on racism."[24]

OR

"*Racism*—a doctrine or teaching without scientific support that claims to find racial differences in character, intelligence, etc., that asserts the superiority of one race over another or others and that seeks to maintain the supposed superiority of a race or races. Any program of racial discrimination, segregation, etc., based on such beliefs—racist."[25]

I contend that racism, as defined by these reliable, authoritative, acceptable sources of the English language, can be said to be the right of one group to dominate the other (group) based on a false assumption or belief (lacking scientific proof) that psychocultural traits and capacities are determined by biological race and that races differ decisively. These differences being inherent in character, intelligence, morality, etc., make one race superior to other races. It is this imagined superiority that gives them the right to rule over others. It is this imagined superiority that gives

---

23.   *Random House Dictionary, Second Edition, Unabridged 1987.*
24.   *Webster's Third New International Dictionary, Unabridged.*
25.   *Webster's New World Dictionary. Updated 1994 Edition.*

the group the power to execute a policy system of government based on this doctrine of assumption. Racism therefore is a political, social, and economic system of domination and exploitation.

Racism is not segregation. It is not discrimination. It is not prejudice or bias. By themselves, these terms can be used to describe, clarify, or enhance situations. For example, boys and girls are sometimes segregated in certain religious institutions; he/she has discriminating taste; he/she has a bias against grapes with seeds; the judge was prejudicial in his proceedings. However, when these terms are combined, used, implemented, and made into law, then racial discrimination, racial segregation, racial bigotry, racial bias become tools for economic, political, social, exploitation and oppression solely for gain and benefit of the dominate group in power. Failure to observe or obey these (man made) laws by the dominated group can result in harsh consequences, prison or death. Look at history.

Although the dominated group or individual members of the group within the society can segregate, discriminate, be prejudiced or biased, make a racist statement, commit racist acts, or even riot, it is not racism. Rather it is a reaction to political, economic exploitation, and social oppression in which the dominated group can find no immediate recourse or relief. The dominated group lack the collective power, the organized will of the community, to be racist. They are powerless to implement, execute economic, political or social policies based on the beliefs of the group in an ongoing and consistent basis. Racism as practiced by the dominating group, however, is *systemic*. It is ongoing. Racism is a group dynamic. The members of the dominating group participate, contribute, receive financial rewards, benefits, privileges, and status from the maintenance of a false belief and assumption of racial superiority that gives them the right to rule over other human beings. This participation and reception of benefits can be direct or indirect, willing or unwilling, voluntary or involuntary. Even though an individual in the dominate group may or may not express an opposing opinion, the fact that the effect of the dominating groups' action demeans, belittles, dehumanizes, and exploits other human beings makes them participants in the system. Therefore, any individual who is a member of the dominating group can be called a racist. In America the racists call themselves white, members of the Caucasian race.

II

Racism is a Disease

Racism Is a Thought Disorder— A Personality Disorder A Mental Illness

Thus far, this book, by definition and a brief history (His story) demonstrates that racism is a system of beliefs, doctrines, and policies executed politically through government in our society, based on assumptions without basis in scientific fact. The system upon which institutional slavery was legalized is the product of irrational thinking. The racist and his behavior in America meet the criteria for 301.81, a narcissistic personality disorder according to the *DSM-IV, Fourth Edition** (*see exhibits 1 & 2).* Irrational thinking in clinical terms is deemed a thought disorder according to the *DSM-IV**, the *Encyclopedic Dictionary of Psychology*, the *Psychiatric Dictionary*, and the clinical book on alcohol, drug, and other substance abuses, *Loosening the Grip.*

*   (Author's note) Diagnostic and Statistical Manual of Mental Disorders, DSM-IV, Fourth Edition, replaced by DSM-IV-TR (Text Revision), Fourth Edition, had not been published when this paper was written in June, 1994. However these criteria notations and definitions remain the same in the DSM-IV-TR. See author's note, page 38.

Disease Model

The *DSM-IV** states that the term psychotic has historically received a number of different definitions, none of which has achieved universal acceptance. The narrowest definition of psychotic is restricted to delusions or prominent hallucinations, with hallucinations occurring in the absence of insight into their pathological nature. Finally, the term has been defined conceptually as a loss of ego boundaries or a gross impairment in reality testing.

In a psychotic disorder due to general medical condition and in a substance-induced psychotic disorder regarding 291.5, alcohol, with delusions, psychotic refers to delusions or only those that are not accompanied by insight. Finally, in delusion disorder, regarding 297.1, and shared psychotic disorder, regarding 297.3, psychotic is equivalent to delusional (see exhibits 2 & 3).

Continuing according to the *DSM-IV**, "the characteristic symptoms of schizophrenia involve a range of cognitive and emotional dysfunctions that include perception, inferential thinking, language and communication, behavioral monitoring, affect fluency, and productivity of thought and speech, hedonic capacity, volition and drive, and attention. No single symptom is pathognomonic of such schizophrenia; the diagnosis involves the recognition of a constellation of signs and systems associated with impaired occupational or social functioning. It continues to state that schizophrenia involves dysfunction in one or more major areas of functioning (e.g., interpersonal relations, work or education or self-care) (criterion B)."

Racism Is a Thought Disorder
A Psychosis
Psychosis: Self-inflammatory Behavior
Changes in DA in Synapse
Schizophrenia

The Encyclopedic Dictionary of Psychology, edited by Harre and Lamb, describes the following, "THOUGHT DISORDER—This term is

---

*   *(Author's note) Diagnostic and Statistical Manual of Mental Disorders, DSM-IV, Fourth Edition, replaced by DSM-IV-TR (Text Revision), Fourth Edition, had not been published when this paper was written in June, 1994. However these criteria notations and definitions remain the same in the DSM-IV-TR. See author's note, page 38.*

employed to describe four types of abnormality in thinking: the form of thought (the way in which thoughts are linked together by logical associations), the possession of thought (the feeling that one's thoughts are not one's own), the content of thought (delusions and other related morbid ideas), and the stream of thought in which the speed and abundancy of thoughts is abnormal. The term is also sometimes used in a narrow sense, restricted to formal thought disorder. This includes phenomenon such as thought blocking (a feeling that thoughts have come to a certain stop), flight of ideas, and a general loosening of associations. The latter may be so severe that the result is totally incoherent speech.

Thought disorder has been classified in a variety of ways, none entirely satisfactory. There have also been a range of explanatory theories. "Thought disorder is characteristic of *Schizophrenia, Mania and organic mental state and a precise description of its nature has diagnostic significance.*"[26]

The Encyclopedia of Psychology, Second edition, edited by R.J. Corsini describes the following: *"Psychotic thought disturbances* are usually accompanied by symptoms of delusion, where false beliefs of persecution of *megalomania* predominate; and hallucinations, where the organism generates its own stimulation in any or all sensory modalities. Though these thought disturbances are serious in their own right, they are generally attached to other types of pathological behavior such as delusion, dementia and schizophrenia.

Schizophrenia is an example of a psychogenic thought disorder. In concert with the thought disorder, there are psychological changes such as decrease in the size of the heart, decrease in the volume of the blood flow, decrease in systemic blood pressure, substantial vasconstruction, and the loss of many sensory signs. Schizophrenic's thought disorder seems to demonstrate a conscious sacrifice of physical and emotional life for some alternative "cocooned" existence for the perceived welfare of others. The thought disorder seems to direct an 'escape for survival' as shown by a continued downward adjustment of functioning in an irrational struggle to stay alive. There is withdrawal from social contact and emotional involvement, as well as regression toward a lower level of intellectual function. This exclusive nihilistic thought disturbance exhibits itself in paranoid, catatonic, hebephrenic, and

---

26. The Encyclopedic Dictionary of Psychology, edited by Ron Harre and Roger Lamb. MIT Press, 1983

simple types. Although schizophrenia is characterized by various levels of severity, more severe cases will show oscillation between stupor and excitement."[27]

Disorders Involving Psychosis

Kinney and Leaton, in *Loosening the Grip,* state that, "*Psychosis* refers to a disorder of perceptions with frequent associated disturbances in function. The term psychotic is often used to describe the thinking of clients with schizophrenia. While psychosis is a symptom that may be associated with a variety of psychiatric disorders, including substance use disorders, it is often prominent in schizophrenic disorders. The schizophrenic disorders are a group of chronic fluctuating disturbances that are among the most incapacitating of the mental disorders. These are also referred to as 'thought disorders.' These disorders have a biochemical basis but are subject to environmental influences"[28] (see exhibits 3 & 4).

Encyclopedia of Psychology, Second Edition Vol. 2 edited by, Corsini states the following, "*Psychosis*—(1) profound disorganization disorganization of mind, personality, or behavior that results from an individual's inability to tolerate the demands of his social environment whether because of the enormity of the imposed stress or because of primary inadequacy or acquired ability of his organism, esp. in regard to the CNS or because of combinations of these factors and that may be manifested by disorders of perception, thinking, or by criminality or by any combination of these—distinguished from neurosis; compare insanity. (2) Extreme mental unrest of an individual or of a social group, especially in regard to situational factors of grave import.<war) mas >—compare hysteria 2; syn. see insanity (see exhibits 2, 3 & 4).

The term *psychosis* is commonly used to denote serious disorder of mental functioning, as in organic affective or schizophrenic psychosis. Beyond this, there is no general agreement on its usage. In some context, it denotes a disturbance that has features of a clear-cut illness (for example, a psychosis resulting from thyroid underactivity as opposed to a condition

---

[27]   *Encyclopedia of Psychology,* Second edition, Edited R. J. Corsini. John Wiley & Sons, 1994.

[28]   Kinney, J. & Leaton, G., *Loosening the Grip ,* McGraw-Hill

that could be seen to evolve from natural reactions and personality characteristics that would be termed *neurosis*. In other contexts, it specifies a mental state encompassing delusions and hallucinations of loss of insight. Psychoanalysts view the mental content of psychosis as deriving from the unconscious id that erupts unchecked into consciousness. Jaspers draws a distinction between mental phenomena that can be understood emphatically and others (encountered in the psychosis) that are accessible only to causal explanations"[29] (see exhibit 4).

Neurosis: Organic Mental State
Mental Illness

Encyclopedia of Psychology, Second Edition Vol. 2 edited by, Corsini states, "The following characteristics of the medical model have been noted by Karchin: Mental illnesses are diseases having etiology, course and outcome; they-have organic bases; like physical ailments, there is an underlying state with surface symptoms; cure depends primarily on medical intervention; and the disease process is within the person.

Mood Disorders—mood and emotions are what you show and how you show it.

Psychosis—refers to a disorder of perceptions with frequent associated disturbances in function.

Neurosis—any of various mental functional disorders characterized by anxiety, compulsions, phobias, depression, dissociations, etc.

Psychosis—a major mental disorder in which the personality is very seriously disorganized and contact with reality is usually impaired: Psychoses are of two sorts, a) functional, characterized by lack of apparent organic cause, and principally of the schizophrenic, paranoid or manic-depressive type, and b) organic characterized by a pathological organic condition such as brain damage or disease, metabolic disorders—syn. insanity.

Megalomania—1. a mental disorder characterized by illusions of grandeur, wealth, power, etc.; 2. a passion for, or for doing, big things. 3. a tendency to exaggerate"[29] (see exhibits 1 & 2).

---

[29] *Encyclopedia of Psychology,* Second Edition Vol. 2. Corsini, R. J .Ed, John Wiley & Sons, 1994

III

Applying Alcoholics Anonymous Principles to The Disease of Racism Comparisons/Similarities to Alcoholism

Based on the background of history (His story) on the North American continent as presented, I have come to the conclusion that racism, as it has evolved in every nook and cranny of the American dream, is a disease, a mental illness. It affects people of color, in particular those descendants of the Africans brought to these shores against their will and given the name slave, Negroes, coloreds, black, and now calling themselves African Americans. It is a primary disease, like alcoholism. Similar to alcoholism, it is a primary disease that has proven to have immediate consequences for the victims, which in time, if not treated or arrested, will prove fatal to the victims (see exhibits 3 & 4).

The victimizers continue to act in a racist manner through their own self-denial, rationalization of behavior and transference of anger to their victims, *causing the victims to think that they are the victimizers*. The victims should seek help for themselves and their families, even though the racist (like the alcoholic) is still active. The racists' behavior has continued to develop over a period of four hundred years. Like the significant other whose life is affected by the alcoholic, I am suggesting that the victims of racism, blacks and other peoples of color in America, apply the principles of Alcoholics Anonymous (AA) to heal themselves and their families. Their lives, like those of the victims of the alcoholic's dysfunctional behavior, have been made dysfunctional as well. Racism, like alcoholism, leaves the victim and the victimizers spiritually bankrupt. AA, Alcoholics Anonymous, has dramatically changed the lives of many alcoholics and transformed the lives of their families and others.

Alcoholics Anonymous (AA) was founded by Bill W., an alcoholic, for alcoholics. AA has helped millions of people whose lives were controlled by this disease. By attending AA meetings, they learned to apply the Serenity Prayer, the twelve steps, the twelve traditions, and slogans to their lives. Applying these AA principles and the Serenity Prayer in regular meetings has produced spectacular results, restoring lives of people who have been affected by this physically, emotionally, psychologically, and spiritually crippling disease.

Alcoholics Anonymous proved so effective that the victims of alcoholic behavior began to apply the AA principles to their own lives. Lois W., the wife of Bill W., founded Al-Anon. Al-Anon was established for people whose lives are affected by another person's excessive drinking, most often a loved one. In the Al-Anon program, they learned that they are able to improve the quality of their lives, even though the alcoholic is still drinking. They learn that they cannot control or stop the alcoholic's drinking. In their attempts to do so, they learn that they become enablers and codependents responsible for the alcoholic's dysfunctional behavior. They become victims to be manipulated by the alcoholic.

The alcoholic in his/her sickness becomes so skillful at transference and countertransference, in which the victim (enabler or codependent) is made to feel guilty and responsible for the alcoholic's behavior. The victim is made to feel like a victimizer. They learn that by attending Al-Anon meetings and using the AA principles in their lives, they can lovingly detach from the alcoholic by allowing him/her to suffer the consequences of their own dysfunctional behavior. They, the victims, learn to stop trying to protect or shield them, the victimizer or the alcoholic, from the consequences of their behavior. They learn instead to keep the focus on their own selves and not on the alcoholic.

Applying the AA principles has been so successful that people have begun applying AA principles to other areas of their lives that are out of control. The twelve-step program and its principles developed by AA and Al-Anon have now been adopted, adapted, and used by other groups to address other dysfunctional behaviors. Some of the groups are Narcotics Anonymous, Gamblers Anonymous, Debtors, and Overeaters Anonymous. The principles of AA, the twelve steps, the twelve traditions, and the slogans have transformed lives in every aspect, socially, psychologically, economically, and most clearly, spiritually.

Suggested Alcoholics Anonymous (AA) Meeting Format for the Victims of Racism

I am suggesting that discussions on racism by the victims be taken one step further by using the AA and Al-Anon twelve-step meeting format. The process would begin in the same manner as the typical AA gathering in a non-threatening environment. Utilizing the AA principles to combat racism in a positive way would involve transposing the key words in the steps, traditions, and slogans. For example: *"Alcoholism [racism] is a disease that we did not cause, we cannot cure, we cannot control and neither can they (the racists)."* This would be followed by the Serenity Prayer, "God Grant Me the Serenity to Accept the Things I Cannot Change, the Courage to Change the Things I Can and the Wisdom to know the Difference."

This is followed by reading the twelve steps and then the twelve traditions aloud. Substitute the word racist or racism where alcohol is indicated. With the slogans visible, participants share experiences of racial incidents, past or present, and how it made them feel. Many African Americans and other victims of color who have had experiences with other twelve-step programs will find this concept, I believe, familiar and comfortable. There is a tendency whenever African Americans gather, no matter what our socioeconomic status, eventually we engage in discussions about them (the racists and racism) and what is being done to us.

Enabling the Racist

Instead of helping the alcoholic, the enabler/codependent eventually takes on the same characteristics of the alcoholic—anger, low self-esteem, and resentment—and eventually become subject to the same effects that would eventually be fatal to the alcoholic. The victims, the enablers/codependents, become victims to a disease that is progressive, unless there is intervention. The affected person, the victim, becomes physically, emotionally, psychologically, and spiritually ill as stated earlier. Like the victims in Al-Anon, the victims of racism need a program for every day—"one day at a time"—to relieve the stress and strain of living. They can begin to learn how to apply the AA principles to their lives and to lovingly detach from the racist and begin to put the focus on themselves. Therefore I propose that the victims of racism, since it is very obvious from a historical point of view that the racist and racism will not stop or go away, begin to apply the AA and the Al-Anon principles to their lives.

In AA, Al-Anon, and other twelve-step programs, there is conference-approved literature. The victims of racism should have approved literature to read when they gather in fellowship. Three books are suggested as required reading for a start. They are Booker T. Washington's *Up From Slavery*, Marcus Garvey's *Philosophy and Opinions of Marcus Garvey*, and W. E. B. Du Bois's *The Souls of Black Folks*. The writing, educational, political, and economic philosophy of these three men in particular contributed to the early uplifting of the African people. Their contributions and influence along with other famous Black men and woman are in evidence today—the Black Middle Class.

W. E. B. Du Bois in his essay "The Talented Tenth," published in 1903, advocated for educating and developing a small group of well-educated blacks who would reach back and raise up their less fortunate brothers and sisters. Booker T. Washington and his early leadership at the Tuskeegee Institute was the foundation that sent thousands of young men and women back into mostly Southern communities to inspire, teach, and lead by example. So inspirational was Washington's book, *Up From Slavery*, that it inspired Marcus Garvey, an African from the Caribbean, to found a school in Jamaica based on Washington's principles of self-help. He decided to meet with Washington for further consultation and collaboration. The meeting never took place due to Washington's death. However, Marcus Garvey went on to found the Negro Improvement Association (NIA) that recruited, organized, and inspired tens of thousands of Blacks in the early twentieth century. His philosophy instilled racial pride and links to Africa, a moving force for Black Nationalism today.

W. E. B. Du Bois was the moving force behind the Niagara Movement, which is now the National Association for the Advancement of Colored People (NAACP). Du Bois would later become a prime mover in the Pan-African Movement that played a leading role in the decolonization of Africa. Reading, studying, and learning about these and other outstanding achievements and accomplishments of the Africans, men and women, on the American Continent, despite the impact and the trauma of racism, could prove to be uplifting and motivational, indeed healing.

IV

Why Racism Should Be of Concern to Clinicians and Individuals Who Aspire to Counsel Others in the Areas of Alcohol, Drug, and Other Substance Abuse/Addictions

Working as a trained substance abuse/addictions counselor, case manager in homeless shelters, chaplain, and relapse prevention specialist, it is my strong belief that racism, like alcoholism must be treated as a disease, a mental illness, a thought disorder. It is a psychosis that through reinforcement over 400 years, has developed into schizophrenia and other mental disorders as defined in the *DSM-IV*.* The racist has clearly demonstrated a personality disorder that can be identified. The racist, according to the *DSM-IV-TR*, fulfills the diagnostic criteria for 301.81, narcissistic personality disorder, a malaise that has left many inhabitants living in America mentally and spiritually drained. Both the victims and victimizers' behaviors are clearly dysfunctional (see exhibits 1-4).

For example, the National Survey on Drug Use and Health (NSDUH) in 2005 reported that there are approximately 16 million heavy drinkers in the United States. What every clinician learns and knows is that alcoholic behavior affects the lives of at least *ten* people in their life. The mathematics of the problem reveals a startling conclusion. Sixteen million heavy drinkers multiplied by 10 equals 160 million people in the United States affected by alcoholic behavior. The NSDUH reported in the same year that there

---

* (Author's note) Diagnostic and Statistical Manual of Mental Disorders, DSM-IV, Fourth Edition, replaced by DSM-IV-TR (Text Revision), Fourth Edition, had not been published when this paper was written in June, 1994. However these criteria notations and definitions remain the same in the DSM-IV-TR.

were 19.6 million illegal drug users. Using the same multiple of 10, there are 196 million people whose lives are affected by illegal drug users.

Combining the alcohol and illegal drug statistics

16 million alcoholics	160 million lives affected
<u>19.6 million illegal drug users</u>	<u>196 million lives affected</u>
35.6 million alcoholic/illegal drug use	356 million lives affected

Aware that this number of affected lives exceeds the last US census of 310 million Americans. It is possible for persons with a drinking or drug problem may have another mental illness as a direct result of drug or alcohol use for instance, schizophrenia or a bipolar disorder, simultaneously. The simultaneous occurrence of two or more illnesses is defined as Comorbidity. Not included in the above are legal prescription drug abusers and other mental disorders. For instance, the National Institute of Mental Health funded the largest detailed survey of the Nation's Mental Health, spending a total of 20 million dollars. The name of the study, *National Comorbidity Survey Replication (NCS-R)*. One of the facts revealed in the 2005 Survey was that "mental disorders are common in the United States and internationally. An estimated 26.2 percent of Americans 18 years and older—about one in four adults—suffer from a diagnosable mental disorder in a given year." The research suggests that America is poised to rank number one globally for mental health disorders.

Racism: A Primary Disease?

Racism and its effects should be taken into serious consideration as a contributing cause of mental illness and relapse when treating African Americans and other peoples of color for substance abuse/addiction, Native Americans in particular. Why? Because after 400 years, the racist, since placing his foot on the American Continent, shows no sign of changing his behavior. Our society remains much the same as it began, directed by a few white men, the majority of whom were WASPs. Although today they are no longer the majority, America remains a society where the white male dominates and rules supreme by domination and aversion based on a thought disorder of superiority and his right to rule. Corporate America in every aspect is a primary example of this power. For instance, out sourcing of major industries and manufacturing jobs overseas. Its historic attempts to destroy the labor movement and even now efforts to cut the collective bargaining power of the unions is well documented. The refusal of big banks to lend to small businesses, the major providers of employment, and failure to re-write or restructure mortgages already backed by the government is an example of corporate greed. These have been a major source of income and financial building blocks for middle class Americans and their children. Millions of them have loss economic status as a result and millions more now face bankruptcy. Billions of dollars pocketed by Corporate CEO's go unchallenged or questioned not even by the most powerful man on the planet, the President of the United States, and hardly a sound from the equally powerful members of Congress. These are some of the prime examples of white male privilege which has always existed from the very beginning of this country. It was incorporated into the by-laws that govern this nation by the "Founding Fathers." John Jay the first supreme court justice said it well, *"Those who own the country should govern it."* Corporate America is today the plantation system of yesterday, with all the same dysfunctions (see exhibits 1 & 2).

When the system has extracted all out of its workers, it discards them like an old dishcloth. The almost total absence of the black male in corporate America is blatantly apparent. The token black males and white females who are admitted must assume the white male profile in order to succeed. The black female, on the other hand, is relegated to clerical positions in great numbers. This racist model functions no matter who is in control. It is behavior that clearly is dysfunctional and fulfills practically all the diagnostic criteria of mental thought disorders found in the *DSM-IV-TR.* When confronted, the racist's rationale of denial and transference of guilt and manipulation is similar to the dysfunctional behavior of the alcoholic (see exhibits 2-4).

It is further felt that the disease concept of racism be seriously studied, researched, and investigated by clinicians involved in the behavioral sciences: psychiatrist, psychologist, social workers, and counselors (see exhibits 3&4). Is racism a contributing cause for relapse and another aspect of treatment to be investigated? Should the shared psychotic disorder (Folie a'Deux) 297.3 listed in the *DSM-IV-TR* be further researched to see how applicable this dysfunction is to African Americans and other peoples of color in America (see exhibits 2 - 4)? Indeed, it is this writer's strong belief, and a challenge for all mental health professionals, especially those in alcohol, drugs and other substance use, that racism be included in the *Diagnostic and Statistical Manual of Mental Disorders, DSM-5*, fifth edition. The *DSM-5* is currently in development and will be published soon. Its purpose, to develop and expand the scientific basis for psychiatric diagnosis and classification.*

Some questions to be considered for further study and research;

1. Is Racism a primary disease? "(see exhibits 3&4).
2. To what extent is racism a contributing factor to these and other mental disorders such as Psychotic Disorders, Mood Disorders, Anxiety Disorders, Somatoform Disorders, Substance Abuse/ Addiction, and Relapse? (see exhibit 4)
3. Does Racism meet the criteria as a specific personality disorder? *(Reference, Antisocial Personality Disorder (PD), 301.7, DSM-IV-TR, Fourth Edition)*

   * (Author's note) Diagnostic and Statistical Manual of Mental Disorders, DSM-IV, Fourth Edition, replaced by DSM-IV-TR (Text Revision), Fourth Edition, had not been published when this paper was written in June, 1994. However these criteria notations and definitions remain the same in the DSM-IV-TR and Section II of the DSM-5 published, May 19 2013. However, in Section III of the DSM-5, an alternative approach was developed for further study to the diagnosis of personality disorders".

4. Should Racism be listed as a mental illness and included in the DSM-5 as a Personality Disorder (PD)? If Not ,why Not? *(Reference, Proposed Revisions for DSM-5 Type and Trait Cross-Walk; DSM-IV-TR Personality Disorder to DSM-5 Type and Trait Cross-Walk)*

V

The Black Church; Source of the Africans Strength Then and Now
The Church of Philadelphia Rises

It would not be fitting to end this book, for me, without acknowledging a debt of gratitude and tribute to the source of our survival as African peoples on the continent of America, the Black Church. In the words of James Baldwin, an outstanding writer, essayist, and social critic, *"It is a miracle that we have survived."* To which this clinician says, "Amen!"

The following commentary gives testimony to the importance of the Black Church's role in the survival of the African then as it does today. C. Eric Lincoln, in his book, *Race, Religion and the Continuing American Dilemma,* writes, *"With fear and trembling . . . as unto Christ. Often when the white man's worship service was over, the black man's might truly begin, for neither his heart nor his private membership was in the white man's church, where he was scorned and demeaned. There was the other church, that invisible institution which met in the swamps and the bayous, and which joined all Black believers in a common experience at a single level of human and spiritual recognition. Deep in the woods and safely out of sight of critical disapproving eyes of the master and overseer, the shouts rolled up and out. The agony so long suppressed burdened the air with sobs and screams and rhythmic moans. God's praises were sung, His mercy enjoined. His justice invoked. There, in the invisible Church, the Black Christian met God on his own terms and in his own way without the white intermediary. That invisible communion was the beginning of the Black Church, the seminal institution which spans most of the history of the Black experience in America. It offers the most accessible key to the complexity and genius of the Black subculture, and it reflects both a vision of the tragedy and an aspect of hope of the continuing American dilemma."[30]*

Lincoln goes on to describe two events that led to the formation of the Black Christian church movement in North America and why. *"In 1787 two events of great historical significance took place in Philadelphia, the city of Brotherly Love. They were in stark contrast to each other in spirit and in their implications for the future of America. The delegates of the Philadelphia Convention gave their approval to the United States Constitution; and a little band of Black Christians led by Richard Allen were pulled from their knees while praying in a segregated gallery in St. George's Methodist Episcopal Church."[31]* Richard Allen was the founder of the African Methodist Episcopal Church (AME) in America. Richard Allen, along with Peter Salem, Absalom Jones, and other African men of spiritual vision became the bulwarks against white racism.

About the second event C. Eric Lincoln writes, *"The Constitution, sadly profaned by three clauses protecting slavery, went on to become the law of the land. Richard Allen and his intrepid band of Black Christians went on to make a different kind of history by institutionalizing the Black Church in America.*

The extraordinary genius of the Christian Religion is exemplified in fact that it has always managed to survive its distortions. For two thousand years the faith has been compromised by countless schisms and isms without succumbing to any of them. Popes, priests, preachers, governments, and private interests have sought from the earliest times to subvert the authority and prestige of the church to private ends. None has enjoyed lasting success. Hence, the strategy of the slavocracy to use Christianity as the linchpin for the institutionalization of slavery and caste in America was ultimately doomed to failure although the failure of the strategy cannot be credited to renouncements of it, early or late. It is not that there have been no prophetic voices in the American Church but at the critical junctures of American history, those voices have always been muted by racism with which we are afflicted. Hence the tragedy of American religion is that it succumbed so early and so completely to the fetish of racism, so clearly in contradiction to the principles by which Christianity claims to be informed.[32]

Lincoln continues *"Capitulation to racial idolatry made God himself, not the African slaves, the principal adversary, for whatever the strategies man may*

---

30. Lincoln, C. Eric, *Race, Religion and the Continuing American Dilemma,* Hill and Wang, New York, 1984, p. 33

31. Ibid, p. 57.

32. Ibid, p. 58.

devise to distain the flesh, only God's lien may lie against the soul. The disdain of the African's body and the labor derived from its possession is a historical fait accompli. But the strategy of American Christianity failed in its effort to make Black Christians a class of spiritual subordinates in concert. For in accepting Christianity in America, the Africans were not necessarily accepting American Christianity. The God they addressed and the faith they knew transcended the American experience. If the white man's religion sacrificed its moral and spiritual validity to the Baal of white supremacy, the Black Church was born of the firm conviction that the racial Baal was a no-god."[33]

My thoughts and reflections on C. Eric Lincoln's narration of the two events, that took place in Philadelphia, in 1787. One wonders if the Apostle St. John writing in the Book of *Revelations*, the last book of the Holy Bible could have been referring to events that would also take place in the city of Philadelphia almost seventeen hundred years later? John the only one of the Apostles not killed because he was a follower of Jesus Christ was in exile on the Island of Patmos. While there, according to his testimony, he was moved by the Holy Spirit to record and send what he saw in a vision to seven churches in Asia Minor. The seven churches were Ephesus, Smyrna, Pergamum, Thyatira, Sardis, Philadelphia and Laodicea. ((Rev. 1: 9 – 12). The Spirit found fault with all but two of the churches. They were the churches of Smyrna and Philadelphia (Rev. 2:8 -11, 3:7- 13).

Is it possible that St. John, in his prophetic vision, could have witnessed the actions of the two Christian groups in Philadelphia, "the City of Brotherly love?" One group, White Christians, dehumanizing their fellow human beings, making them unequal to themselves, reducing them to chattel property through the creation of their man made law and order document, the constitution. This document incorporating the 13 colonies into a "formal union," although legal, was in total violation of the Creator of Law and Order, the commandment of loving God and neighbor. The other group, a tiny band of free African men and women, former slaves, pulled from their knees and put out of the WASP Methodist Church of St. George in Philadelphia for refusing to pray and worship as unequal before the same God. They went on to form their own Christian Protestant Church, the African Methodist Episcopal Church (A.M.E) and later the African Methodist Episcopal Zion Church (A.M.E.Z), founded by, Absalom Jones, that is in existence today.

The Impact of the Black Church in America on the spiritual, cultural, social, and political life of its people is evident today. Its leadership in non

---

33.   Ibid, p. 59.

violent struggle for social justice, civil and human rights here in America has been adapted by peoples in similar circumstances all over the globe. Thousands of tourists, many of them from almost empty churches in Europe, are lining up to attend Sunday morning worship services in the various churches in Harlem. In halting English, often to the amused consternation of church members and parishioners, they hear from the visitors, "gospel, gospel?" One is reminded of John's prophetic voice of encouragement to that small group of Christians in the Church of Philadelphia in Asia Minor.

 "Letter to Philadelphia;

 This is what you must write to the angel of the church in Philadelphia: I am the one who is holy and true, and I have the keys that belonged to David. When I open a door, no one can close it. And when I close a door, no one can open it. Listen to what I say. I know everything you have done. And I place before you an open door that no one can close. You were not very strong, but you obeyed my message and did not deny that you were my followers. Now you will see what I will do with those people who belong to Satan's group. They claim to be God's people, but they are liars. I will make them come and kneel down at your feet. Then they will know that I love you. You obeyed my message and endured. So I will protect you from the time of testing that everyone in the world will go through. I am coming soon. So hold firmly to what you have, and no one will take away the crown that you will be given as your reward. Everyone who wins the victory will be made a pillar in the temple of my God, and they will stay there forever. I will write on each of them the name of my God and the name of his city. It is the New Jerusalem that my god will send down from heaven. I will also write on them my own new name. If you have ears, listen to what the Spirit says to the churches. Rev. 3: 7-13, (The African American Jubilee Edition of the Holy Bible).

 The Word of God and Human Relations; *"He who is not with me is against me, and he who does not gather with me scatters. And so I tell you every one of men's sins and blasphemies will be forgiven, but blasphemy against the Spirit will not be forgiven. And anyone who says a word against the Son of Man will be forgiven; but let anyone speak against the Holy Spirit and he will not be forgiven either in this world or in the next."* Mt: 12: 30-32, The (Jerusalem Bible) *Anyone who says, 'I love God,' and hates his brother, is a liar, since a man who does not love the brother that he can see cannot love God whom has never seen. So this is the commandment that he has given us, that anyone who loves God must also love his brother."* 1 John 4:20, 21 (Jerusalem Bible)

"Your body, you know, is the Temple of the Holy Spirit, who is in you since you received him from God," 1 Corinthians 6:19." If anybody should destroy the Temple of God, God will destroy him, because the temple of God is sacred; and you are that Temple," 1Corinthians 3:17. (Jerusalem Bible)

The following statement is taken from one of many documents reflecting the Roman Catholic Church's teaching on racism;

"IV. Contribution of Christians, in Union with Others, to Promoting Fraternity and Solidarity Among Races;

24. Racial prejudice, which denies the equal dignity of all the members of the human family and blasphemes the Creator, can only be eradicated by going to its roots, where it is formed: in the human heart. It is from the heart that just or unjust behavior is born,(63) according to whether persons are open to God's will-in the natural order and in the Living Word-or whether they close themselves up in those egoisms dictated by fear or the instinct of domination. It is the way we look at others that must be purified. Harboring racist thoughts and entertaining racist attitudes is a sin against the specific message of Christ for whom one's "neighbor" is not only a person from my tribe, my milieu, my religion or my nation: it is every person that I meet along the way."[34] *Brothers and Sisters to Us,* a Pastoral letter, by the US Catholic Bishops, and the Black Catholic Bishops' Pastoral Letter , *"What We have Seen and Heard,"* are other Church documents that address the evil of racism that endures in both society and the Church.

W.E. B Du Bois made the following observation about the 20th century *"The Problem of the Twentieth Century is the problem of the color-line."*[35]

Marcus Garvey offered this advice to the victims of Racism, *"Make your interpretation of Christianity scientific—what it ought to be, and blame no God, blame not the white man for physical conditions for which we ourselves are responsible."*[36]

---

[34] Pontifical Commission Justice and Peace. *The Church and Racism: Toward a more Fraternal Society.* Rome: Vatican, 1988. Print. #24

[35] Du Bois, W.E.B., *The Souls of Black Folk; Three Negro Classics.* New York: Avon, 1965. Print.

[36] Garvey, Amy Jacque, Ed. *Philosophy and Opinions of Marcus Garvey,* Vols. I & II, Atheneum, New York, 1968.

In conclusion it is my hope, indeed my prayer that the racists and the victims of racism seek help by applying Alcoholics Anonymous Principles to the Disease of Racism, until it is stopped, arrested, or undone in the 21st century. Rev. Kenneth L. Radcliffe, Deacon, Founder, The ISAIAH Project 61 & The Criminal "JUST US" Committee.

Bibliography

Historical Sources

Bennett, Lerone, Jr., *Before the Mayflower*, Johnson Publishing Co., Chicago, Ill. Inc.

Berry, Brewton, PhD, *Race Relations-Interaction of Ethnic and Racial Groups,* Houghton Mifflin Company, Boston, Ma. 1951.

Brown, Dee. *Bury My Heart at Wounded Knee.* New York: Owl Books, Henry Holt and Company, 1970. Print

Close, Ellis, *Rage of A Privileged Class,* Harper Collins, 1993.

Davidson, Basil, *The African Slave Trade*, Back Bay Books, Boston, Ma.

Du Bois, W.E.B., *The Souls of Black Folk; Three Negro Classics.* New York: Avon, 1965. Print.

Garvey, Amy Jacque, Ed. *Philosophy and Opinions of Marcus Garvey,* Vols. I & II, Atheneum, New York, 1968.

Gossett, Thomas, *Race: The History of an Idea in America,* Southern Methodist University Press, Dallas, 1963.

Lincoln, C. Eric, *Race Religion and the Continuing American Dilemma,* Hill and Wang, New York, 1984.

Meltzer, Milton, Ed., *In Their Words, A History of the American Negro, 1619–1865; 1865–1916; 1916–1966,* Thomas Y. Crowell Company, New York, 1967.

Washington, Booker, T. *Up from Slavery; Three Negro Classics.* New York: Avon, 1965. Print.

Clinical Sources

Bell, Peter, *Chemical Dependency and the African American,* Hazeldon, 1990.

Corsini, Raymond, J (Ed.). *Encyclopedia of Psychology.* New York: Wiley, 1994. Print.

Corsini, Raymond, J. (Ed.). *International Encyclopedia of Psychiatry, Psychology, Psychoanalysis and Neurology.* Wiley Interscience Publications

American Psychiatric Association. *Diagnostic and Statistical Manual of Mental Disorders. 3rd ed., 4th ed.* Washington, D.C.: American Psychiatric Publishing, Inc.

American Psychiatric Association. *Diagnostic Statistical Manual of Mental Disorders: DSM-4 –TR (Text Revision) 4th ed.* Washington, D.C.: American Psychiatric Publishing, Inc.

American Psychiatric Association. *Diagnostic Statistical Manual of Mental Disorders: DSM-5 Type and Trait cross-Walk).* Washington, D.C.: American Psychiatric Publishing, Inc.

Finnegan, D., McNally, E., *Dual Identities.* Center City, Minn.: Hazeldon, 1987. Print.

Harre, R., Lamb, R. (Eds.). *The Encyclopedic Dictionary,* The MIT Press, 1983.

Johnson, Vernon E., *I'll Quit Tomorrow, A Practical Guide to Alcoholism, Treatment, Revised Edition,* Harper Collins, 1980.

Kovel, Joel *White Racism: A Psychohistory,* Pantheon Books, New York, A division of Random House, 1970

Kinney, J., Leaton, G., *Loosening the Grip: A Handbook Of Alcohol Information.* St. Louis, Mo.: Mosby Year Book, 1991.

McMillin, Chandler Scott, *Don't Help: A Positive Guide to Working with the Alcoholic.* Bantam. Trade Paperback, 1989.

Sandmaier, Marian. *The Invisible Alcoholics, Women and Alcohol, 2nd ed.,* Blue Ridge Summit, Pa.: Tab Books, 1992. Print.

Zimberg, S., Wallace, J., Blume, S. (Eds.). *Practical Approaches to Alcoholism Psychotherapy.* New York: Plenum Press, 1985. Print.

Church Source

Pontifical Commission Justice and Peace. *The Church and Racism: Toward a more Fraternal Society.* Rome: Vatican, 1988. Print.

National Conference of Catholic Bishops. *Brothers and Sisters to Us, U.S. Bishops Pastoral Letter on Racism in Our day.* Ed. U. S Catholic Bishops. Washington, DC: USCCB Publishing, 1979. Print.

Black Catholic Bishops of the United States. *What We Have Seen and Heard, A Pastoral Letter on Evangelization.* Cincinnati: St. Anthony Press, 1984. Print.

Lucas, Lawrence. *Black Priest White Church, Catholics and Racism.* Africa World Press, 1989. Print

A PROTOTYPE OF A RACIST OF THE 18TH & 19TH CENTURY

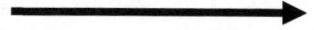

Joel Kovel in his book, *White Racism: A Psychohistory*, takes us into what could have been the mindset of a slaver of the period. He writes. "A particular master-slave relationship developed under specific circumstances of American history. Although there were points of similarity with which other slave systems, much of which remain the subject of active investigation, a basic and characteristically American style emerged as Black slavery developed as an <u>institution.</u> The slaver in effect said to his slave, *'while I own much, much more than my body, you own, not even your body: your body shall be detached from yourself and yourself shall thereby be reduced to subhuman status. And being detached and kept alive, your body shall serve me in many ways: by work on my capitalist plantations to extract the most that can be taken from the land in the cheapest and therefore most rational manner,—as a means to my bodily pleasure—both as nurse to my children and as a female body for sexual use (for my women are somehow deficient in this regard), and as a medium of exchange, salable like any other commodity of exchange along with or separate from the bodies if your family. For in fact you have no family, since a family is a system that pertains to the human being and you are not human. And since I, being a man of the West, value things which are owned above all else, I hold you or rather the owned part of you, your body—in very high regard and wish to retain you as my property forever. On the other hand, since I have a certain horror of what I am doing and since you are the living reminder of this horror and are subhuman, I am horrified by you, disgusted by you, and wish to have nothing to do with you. I wish in fact to be rid of you. And since this set of ideas is inconsistent and will not stand neither the test of reason nor of my better values I am going to distort it, spit it up, and otherwise defend myself against the realization.'*

In practice this schema underwent endless variations. The distillation of this notion was the essence of the American slave system however, and had a reality of its own: it became the basis in culture of the idea of the Black man, and it has consequently become the historical nucleus of our present—day racism."*

---

* Kovel, J., *White Racism: A Psychohistory*, Pantheon Books, New York, Division of Random House, 1970, pp. 18, 19.

- **Diagnostic criteria for 301.81 Narcissistic Personality Disorder**

  A pervasive pattern of grandiosity (in fantasy or behavior), need for admiration and lack of empathy, beginning by early adulthood and present in a variety of contexts, as indicated by five (or more) of the following:

  (1) Has a grandiose sense of self-importance (e.g. exaggerates achievements and talents, expects to be recognized as superior without commensurate achievements)

  (2) Is preoccupied with fantasies of unlimited success, power, brilliance, beauty, or ideal love

  (3) Believes that he or she is "special" and unique and can only be understood by, or should associate with, other special or high status people (or institutions)

  (4) Requires excessive admiration

  (5) Has a sense of entitlement, i.e., unreasonable expectations of especially favorable treatment or automatic compliance with his or her expectations

  (6) Is interpersonally exploitative, i.e. takes advantage of others to achieve his or her own ends

  (7) Lacks empathy: is unwilling to recognize or identify with the feelings or needs of others

  (8) Is often envious of others or believes that others are envious of him or her

  (9) Shows arrogant, haughty behaviors or attitudes

E
X
H
I
B
I
T

1

Megalomania - 1.a mental disorder characterized by illusions of grandeur, wealth, power, etc. 2. a pattern for, or for doing, big things. 3. a tendency to exaggerate

A PSYCHOTIC DISORDER FOR THOSE SLAVES WHO CHOOSE NOT TO REBEL, REMAINED SUBMISSIVE, DOCILE

MANY SLAVES STAYED WITH THEIR MASTER LONG AFTER EMANCIPATION

- **Diagnostic criteria for 297.31 Shared Psychotic Disorder**

  A. A delusion develops in an individual in the context of a close relationship with another person(s), who has an already established delusion.

  B. The delusion is similar in content to that of the person who already has the established delusion.

  C. The disturbance is not accounted for by another Psychotic Disorder (e.g. Schizophrenia) or a Mood Disorder With Psychotic Features and is not due to the direct physiological effects of a substance (e.g. a drug of abuse, a medication, or a general medical condition.

Source: DSM-IV/DSM-IV-TR (see author's note p. 26).

A PROTOTYPE OF A RACIST OF THE 20TH CENTURY

——————————————▶

Our society remains much the same as it began, directed by a few white men, the majority of whom were WASPs. Although today they are no longer the majority, America remains a society where the white male dominates and rules supreme by domination and aversion based on a thought disorder of superiority and the right to rule. Corporate America in every respect is the primary expression of white male dominance and privilege. It is today the plantation system of yesterday, with all the same dysfunctions (see Racism: A Primary Disease? Pp. 36 & 37).

A PSYCHOTIC DISORDER FOR MANY AFRICAN AMERICANS IN THE WORKPLACE?

"Though they struggle to hold their anger in check, even the most successful Blacks find themselves haunted by racial demons." This and the following excerpts are taken from a book entitled "The Rage of a Privileged Class" by Ellis Cose.

"There is an air of frustration (among Black managers) that's just as high now as it was 30 years ago . . . they have an even worse problem (than I did) because they've got MBA's from Harvard. They did all the things you're supposed to do . . . and things are supposed to happen." Darwin Davis, Sr. V. P .Equitable Life Assurance Society.

"Differential Diagnosis
The diagnosis of Shared Psychotic Disorder is made only when the delusion is not due to the direct physiological effects of a substance or a general medical condition. Differential diagnosis is rarely a problem because the history of a close association with the primary case and the similarity of delusions between the two individuals are unique to Shared Psychotic Disorder. In Schizophrenia, Delusional Disorder Schizoaffective Disorder and Mood Disorder with Psychotic Features, there is either no close relationship with a dominant person who has a Psychotic Disorder and shares similar delusional beliefs or, if there is such a person, the psychotic symptoms usually precede the onset of any shared Psychotic disorder, but the delusions do not disappear when the individual is separated from the primary case. In such a situation, it is probably appropriate to consider another Psychotic Disorder Diagnosis."*

* Source: <u>DSM-IV-TR® Handbook of Differential Diagnosis</u>

- **Diagnostic criteria for 301.81 Narcissistic Personality Disorder**
  A pervasive pattern of grandiosity (in fantasy or behavior), need for admiration and lack of empathy, beginning by early adulthood and present in a variety of contexts, as indicated by five (or more) of the following:
  - (1) has a grandiose sense of self-importance (e.g. exaggerates achievements and talents, expects to be recognized as superior without commensurate achievements)
  - (2) is preoccupied with fantasies of unlimited success, power, brilliance, beauty, or ideal love
  - (3) believes that he or she is "special" and unique and can only be understood by, or should associate with, other special or high status people (or institutions)
  - (4) requires excessive admiration
  - (5) Has a sense of entitlement, i.e., unreasonable expectations of especially favorable treatment or automatic compliance with his or her expectations
  - 6) is interpersonally exploitative, i.e. takes advantage of others to achieve his or her own ends
  - (7) lacks empathy: is unwilling to recognize or identify with the feelings or needs of others
  - (8) is often envious of others or believes that others are envious of him or her
  - (9) shows arrogant, haughty behaviors or attitudes

EXHIBIT 2

Megalomania - 1.a mental disorder characterized by illusions of grandeur, wealth, power, etc. 2. a pattern for, or for doing, big things. 3. a tendency to exaggerate

BLACK CORPORATE EXECUTIVES

A PSYCHOTIC DISORDER FOR MANY AFRICAN AMERICANS IN THE WORK PLACE?

- **Diagnostic criteria for 297.3 Shared Psychotic Disorder**
  A.   A delusion develops in an individual in the context of a close relationship with another person(s), who has an already established delusion.
  B.   The delusion is similar in content to that of the person who already has the established delusion.
  C.   The disturbance is not accounted for by another Psychotic Disorder (e.g. Schizophrenia) or a Mood Disorder with Psychotic Features and is not due to the direct physiological effects of a substance (e.g. a drug of abuse, a medication, or a general medical condition.

Source: DSM-IV/DSM-IV-TR (see author's note p. 26).

DEFINITION OF ALCOHOLISM*

Alcoholism is a *primary* chronic *disease* with genetic, psychosocial, and environmental factors influencing its development and manifestations. The disease is *often progressive and fatal.* It is characterized by continuous or periodic *impaired control* over drinking, *preoccupation* with the **drug alcohol**, use of **alcohol** despite *adverse consequences*, and distortions in thinking, most notably *denial.*

(SUBSTITUTE THE WORD RACISIM WHEREVER ALCOHOL, ALCOHOLISM OR DRINKING APPEAR)

- **Primary** refers to the nature of **alcoholism** as a disease entity in addition to and separate from other pathophysiologic states which may be associated with it. Primary suggests that **alcoholism,** as an addiction is not a symptom of an underlying disease state.
- **Disease** means an involuntary disability. It represents the sum of the abnormal phenomena displayed by a group of individuals. These phenomena are associated with a specified common set of characteristics by which these individuals differ from the norm, and which places them at a disadvantage.
- **o*ften progressive*** and fatal means that the disease persists over time and that physical, emotional, and social changes are often cumulative and may progress as **drinking** continues. **Alcoholism** causes premature death through overdose, organic complications involving the brain, liver, heart and many other organs, and by contributing to suicide, homicide, motor vehicle crashes, and other traumatic events.
- **Impaired control** means the inability to limit **alcohol use** or to consistently limit on any **drinking** occasion the duration of the episode, the quantity consumed and/or the behavioral consequences of **drinking.**
- **Preoccupation** in association **with alcohol use** indicates excessive, focused attention given to the **drug alcohol**, its effects, and/or its use. The relative value thus assigned to **alcohol** by the individual often leads to a diversion of energies away from important life concerns.
- **Adverse consequences** are **alcohol**-related problems or impairments in such areas as: physical health (e.g. alcohol withdrawal syndromes, liver disease, gastritis, anemia, neurological disorders); psychological functioning (e.g. marital problems and child abuse, impaired social relationships); occupational functioning (e.g. scholastic or job problems); and legal, financial, or spiritual problems.

- d**enial** is used here not only in the psychoanalytic sense of a single psychological defense mechanism disavowing the significance of events, but more broadly to include a range of psychological maneuvers designed to reduce awareness of the fact that **alcohol use** is the cause of an individual's problems rather than a solution to those problems. Denial becomes an integral part of the disease and a major obstacle to recovery.*

A DISEASE MODEL FOR RACISM COMPARISONS/SIMILARITIES TO ALCOHOLISM

E
X
H
I
B
I
T

3

→ *THE DEFINITION FOR ALCHOLISM AND ITS EFFECTS ARE SIMILAR AND ALMOST IDENTICAL TO THE EFFECTS OF RACISM ON THE VICTIMS OF RACISM—AFRICANS, NATIVE AMERICANS AND OTHER PEOPLES OF COLOR.*

OVERVIEW OF ALCOHOLISM: THE FEELING DISEASE

DISEASE: Chemical dependency (**alcoholism** and/or harmful dependence on any mood-altering drug) is a disease. A disease has its own symptoms and is describable

A. **PRIMARY DISEASE**: It is not a secondary symptom of something else.

B. **PROGRESSIVE DISEASE**: The disease gets progressively worse unless intervened with. The person becomes physically, spiritually, emotionally and psychologically more ill.

C. **CHRONIC DISEASE**: There is no cure. Remission from the active phases of the disease must be based on abstinence from **mood-altering chemicals** and an ongoing program of recovery.

D. **FATAL DISEASE**: If the disease is not arrested, the person is at the highest risk for premature death (**alcohol**-related illness, suicide, accidents, etc.

*This definition was prepared by the Joint Committee in Study the Definition and Criteria for the Diagnosis of Alcoholism of the National Council on Alcoholism and Drug Dependence and the American Society of Addiction Medicine. It was approved by the Board of Directors of NCADD on 3 February, 1990 and the Board of Directors of ASAM on 25 February, 1990.

- **ALCOHOLISM IS A THOUGHT DISORDER, A PSYCHOSIS**

- **RACISM IS A THOUGHT DISORDER, A PSYCHOSIS**

  - **RACISM IS A GROUP DYNAMIC**

    - **RACISM IS SYSTEMIC**

Racism is dangerous to the health of African Americans and other peoples of color.

"But the West is extraordinary in that it has held for centuries that the summum bonum of life on earth is the expansion of the self through its acquisition of property. On the other hand, the West, which was to convulse the globe in its search for material acquisitions, has never really been happy with its desire for property. Nowadays the whole process—desire for and horror of acquisition—has, without losing its basic force been rationalized and made abstract: this has been the consistent direction of our history." Kovel, J., *White Racism: A Psychohistory* (see exhibit 1).

"The white man made us many promises – more than I can remember, but he never kept but one: he promised to take our land—and he took it" Red Cloud. *Bury My Heart At Wounded Knee,* Dee Brown, 1970.

THE IMPACT OF ALCOHOL DRUGS AND RACISM ON THE POOR IN BLACK URBAN AMERICA

These are some excerpts taken from comments made by Henry Cisneros, Secretary of Housing Urban Development (HUD) on NBC "Meet the Press" Sunday December 26, 1993.

"After a string of urban riots that took place across Urban America—Newark, New York, Detroit, Watts—a federal commission was formed. It was headed by Otto Kerner, former Governor of Illinois. The final *conclusion of the commission's report in 1968 was "America is moving toward two societies, one Black, one White . . ."* He *said that this was largely responsible for the frustrations that led to the violence in many inner cities."*

"*Despite tremendous gains for many Americans including Afro-Americans . . . for many (urban dwellers) life is a lot worse."*

"*The plight of the cities is worse today than it was 25 years ago when a presidential commission declared that urban America was in crisis because of racial division . . ."*

"*We have neglected the cities over the past generation and, in addition, we have seen the rise of racism (becoming) fashionable again . . ."*

" *. . . the combination of drugs, a lack of jobs, racial strife, and general decline in the quality of life has made conditions worse than . . . when the Kerner Commission wrote that 'the cities were in crisis."*

IMPACT ON MANY BLACK CORPORATE EXECUTIVES

I think it's very difficult once we have achieved, and we have good educations, and we know we're good . . Nobody wants to be perceived as being a victim of racism or prejudice. It hurts. It hurts deeply." Ella Louise Bell, Asst. Professor: Sloan School of Management, MIT.

"*When the system has extracted all out of its workers, it discards them like an old dishcloth. The almost total absence of the Black male in Corporate America is blatantly apparent. The token black males and white females who are admitted must assume the white male profile in order to succeed. The black female, on the other hand, is relegated to clerical positions in great numbers. This racist model functions no matter who is in control. It is behavior that clearly is dysfunctional and fulfills all the diagnostic criteria of mental thought disorders found in the DSM-IV-TR. When confronted, the racist's rationale of denial and transference of guilt and manipulation is similar to that of the behavior of an alcoholic."* Kenneth L. Radcliffe, Deacon

SUGGESTED SOURCES
FOR FURTHER RESEARCH AND STUDY

This author recommends that these sources be used when considering these questions for further study and research by mental health and medical professionals, i.e. psychiatrists, psychologists, social workers, alcohol and other substance use counselors.

DSM-IV-TR® Diagnostic and Statistical Manual of Mental Disorders, 4th Edition, The American Psychiatric Association, American Psychiatric Publishing, Inc.

DSM-IV-TR® Handbook of Differential Diagnosis
Michael B. First, M.D., Allen Frances, M.D., Harold Alan Pincus, M.D. 4th Ed. by the American Psychiatric Association, American Psychiatric Publishing, Inc.

1. To what extent is racism a contributing factor to these disorders?

Aggressive Behavior, Anxiety, Avoidance Behavior, Behavior Problems in a Child or Adolescent, Catatonia, Changes in Appetite or Unusual Eating Behavior, Delusions, Depressed Mood, Disorganized or Unusual Speech, Distractibility, Elevated or Irritable Mood, Hallucinations, Hypersomnia, Impulsivity, Insomnia, Memory Impairment, Pain, Panic Attacks, Physical Complaints or Irrational Anxiety About Appearance, Poor School Performance, Psychomotor Retardation, Self-Mutilation, Sexual Dysfunction, Suicidal Ideation or Attempt, Presumed Etiology, Mental Disorders Due to a General Medical Condition, Mental Disorder Due to Substance Use, Mental Disorder Due to Stress, Post Traumatic Stress Syndrome (not diagnosed, untreated for the descendants of the Africans brought to the Americas and other peoples of color.)

2. Is Racism a Primary Cause?

3. Should Racism be designated as a Primary Disease, a Mental Illness, Personality Disorder (PD) or both?

4. Should Racism be included in the soon to be published DSM—5, Fifth Edition, as a Personality Disorder (PD)? If not, why not? (see page 38)